PET THERAPY

I0421206

LEARN HOW TO USE PET THERAPY TO CONTROL YOUR MENTAL ILLNESS

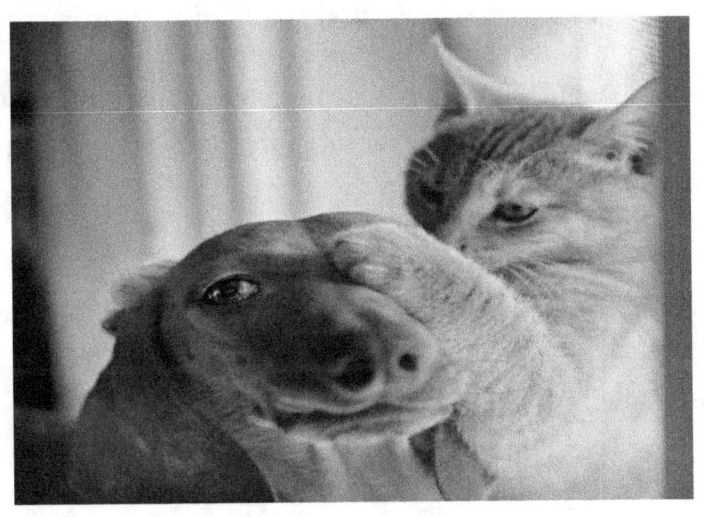

By Patricia A Carlisle

Introduction

I want to thank you and congratulate you for choosing the book, *"PET THERAPY: How to Use Pet Therapy to Control Your Mental Illness"*.

Pet Therapy is a guided interaction between an individual and a trained animal. It also involves the animal's handler. The purpose of pet therapy is to help a patient recover, or cope with a health problem or a mental disorder. Pet therapy also is called animal-assisted therapy.

Dogs and cats are the animals most commonly used in pet therapy. However, fish, guinea pigs, horses, and other animals that meet screening criteria can be used. The type of animal chosen depends on the therapeutic goals of a patient's treatment plan.

Pet therapy, is sometimes confused with animal-assisted activities. Pet therapy is a formal, structured set of encounters. These meetings are planned to help patients reach specific goals in their treatment or progress.

Thanks again for choosing this book, I hope you enjoy it!

Patricia A. Carlisle, MSW, CBT

Patricia Carlisle- A Master Social Worker and a Cognitive Behavioral Therapist (CBT) gives out an expression of how important it is for an individual to take into consideration the concept of self-assessment to know what human, technical and conceptual skills they posses to perform or to achieve what they desire, or to deal with everyday life. However, every particular group of people has their own unique set of ideas, traditions and events including the frame of mind according to which people perform but there are many who faces problems and fail to maintain a healthy mind set affecting their behaviors and performance to those around them.

> People like Patricia Carlisle are among those who have felt this urge of serving people and helping them out of their mental crisis towards a healthy life. She has experienced some close encounters in her personal life regarding mental health issues in her family and friends that has encouraged her to pursue this as her career.

Currently Patricia Carlisle is serving as a Certified On-Line Cognitive Behavioral Therapist with an extensive 15years of experience using Cognitive-Behavior Therapy Techniques. She envisions a world where everyone gets mental health treatment with no mental health stigma and to make it real she has already set up her own Holistic Measure Online Comprehensive Behavioral Healthcare Company after retiring from The Nord Center in The Partial Hospitalization Program (PHP) Dept for 5 years and Murtis H. Taylor Mental Health Center as a mental health counselor, psychological support technician and case manager for 10 years to emulsify her skills more professionally. Along with this, she has wrote down her passion as a clinician in 25 or more short books to help individuals and families get their life back, freeing them of the restraints of negative thinking, anxiety and depression by using different approaches. She is highly appreciated among her clients for her flexibility and professionalism of dealing with them graciously.

To reach her, make use of her direct website address: http://therapist2013.wix.com/e-therapy . As she is ready to inspire hope and contribute to health and well-being by providing the best online health care through comprehensive practice, education and research.

TABLE OF CONTENT

Chapter 1

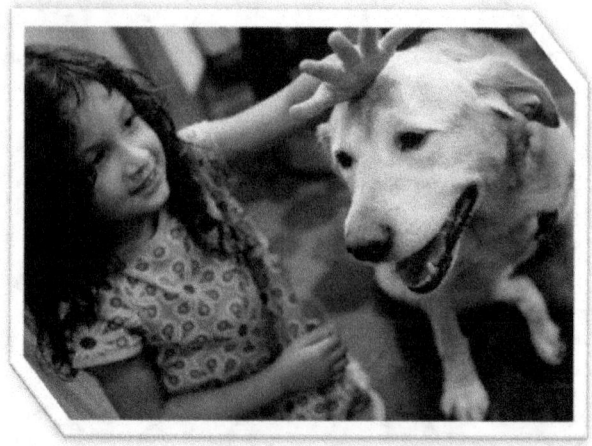

PET THERAPY

Research shows that visiting with a pet can reduce stress symptoms, lower blood pressure temporarily, increase sensory stimulation, and even lengthen a person's life expectancy. Pet therapy is a general term that encompasses many therapeutic activities involving animals as companions, or occasional visitors to the sick, elderly, or mentally ill. Because animals provide unconditional acceptance, pet therapy can be comforting, and can also distract the sick, or the aged from their illnesses or problems.

In areas that are often sterile and lonely, such as hospitals or nursing homes, a pet therapy program can bring screened animals and human volunteers to make visits. These visits can be soothing to the patients or residents, because people tend to be nurturing around animals. When participating in pet therapy, some patients recall fond memories about their own pets. These types of visits are shown to positively affect disposition, and increase social interaction among patients and residents.

Other research has shown that heart patients who either own a pet, or are paired with a pet following discharge from the hospital tend to heal faster, and survive longer. Most likely this is due to the combination of a sense of purpose, and the fact that having a pet can lower stress. The pet does not have to be a dog or cat; it can be a rabbit, fish, parakeet, or other animal.

Many pet therapy programs exist to train, coordinate, and place pets that have been behaviorally and medically screened in schools, medical centers, and homes for the elderly, and troubled teenagers. Pet therapy can have a positive effect on a resident or patient's physical health, as well as on his or her emotional health by reducing loneliness, and creating a sense of purpose. Some animals in a pet therapy program may have specific task, such as "listening' to a patient as he or she has a psychological counseling session, or fetching a ball for a patient who is receiving physical therapy following a stroke. In other pet therapy situations, a pet and volunteer may just visit a hospital, or assisted living so that residents or patients may pet, interact, or play with the animal.

If you own a calm, friendly animal that would make a good pet companion, search the internet for organizations that seek volunteers, or contact a university's school of veterinary medicine for information. The Delta Society is one such international, non-profit, human service organization, that providers companion animals, and also trains volunteers, and screens animals for participation in pet therapy programs.

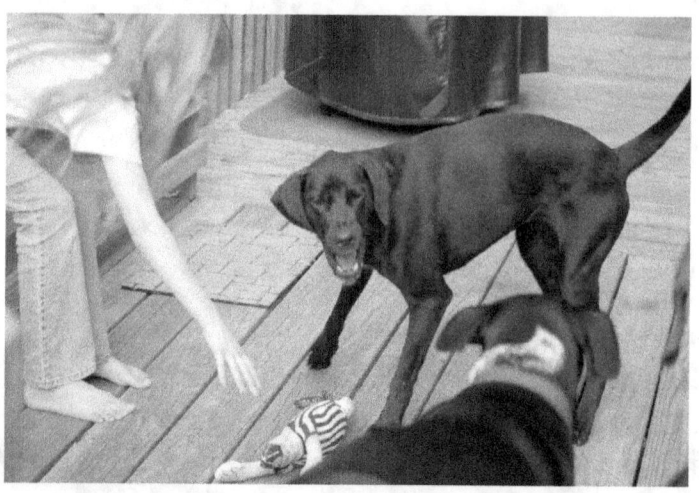

Chapter 2

BENEFITS OF PET THERAPY

Its well-known (and scientifically proven) that interaction with a gentle, friendly pet has significant benefits.

Physical Health:

Lowers blood pressure.

Improves cardiovascular health.

Releases endorphins (oxytocin) that have a calming effect.

Diminishes overall physical pain.

The act of petting produces an automatic relaxation response, reducing the amount of medication some folks need.

Mental Health:

Lifts spirits and lessens depression.

Decreases feelings of isolation and alienation.

Encourages communication.

Provides comfort.

Increases socialization.

Reduces boredom.

Lowers anxiety.

Helps children overcome speech and emotional disorders.

Creates motivation for the client to recover faster.

Reduces loneliness.

Reading: (PAWS for Reading)

Helps children focus better.

Improves literacy skills.

Provides non-stressful, non-judgmental environment.

Increases self-confidence, reduces self-consciousness.

In Physical Therapy:

Increases joint movement, and improves recovery time.

Maintains or increases motor skills.

Provides motivation to move more, stretch farther, exercise longer.

Chapter 3

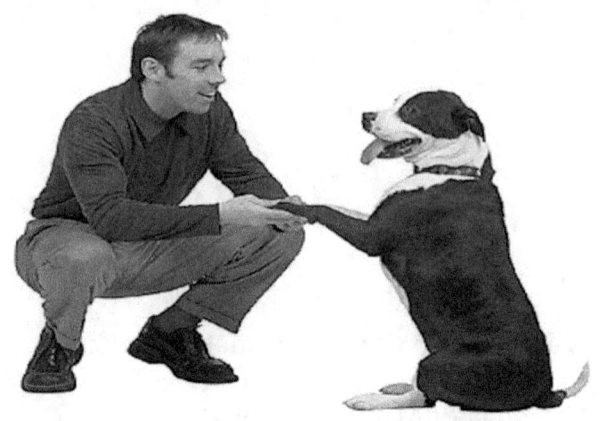

How to Get a Pet Therapy Certification

While any we'll-behaved animal can provide some comfort. and companionship to the sick elderly. and other people in need, getting a certification for you and your pet means you'll be able to do it in more formal settings, such as nursing homes and hospitals. The process for certifying an animal therapy team involves passing an evaluation, but depending on the organization you might have other steps to follow.

Research Organizations:

Before you decide on an organization, research your options, and find one that's well-respected, and recognized by other animal organizations. For example, the American Kennel Club recognizes certifications form Therapy Dogs Incorporated, Therapy Dogs International, Pet Partners, Love on a Leash, and Bright and Beautiful Therapy Dogs. The American Society for the Prevention of Cruelty to Animals, meanwhile, recommends Pet Partners, which certifies dogs as well as cats, rabbits, and other pets. Find out which organization offer a chapter near you, and ask about the cost of certification. Read the organizations' FAQs to find out whether you'll have any conflicts by pursuing one certification or another. Therapy Dogs International, for example, doesn't allow members to register with more than one organization.

Your Animal's Temperament:

A big part of gaining certification depends on the temperament of your pet. Generally, your pet needs to be a "model citizen" that doesn't have a history of biting, growling, or lashing out at humans or other animals. If your pet has a short fuse, he's probably not a good fit for animal therapy. You will need to have sufficient animal handling skills to control your pet, and he should be potty trained.

Pre-Evaluation Activities:

Depending on the organization, you may have to attend a training session for humans, or a pet obedience class as part of the certification process. Pet Partners, for example, has its human candidates attend an animal handler course as one of the first steps in the process. Therapy Dogs International doesn't have a similar requirement, thought it does recommend its dogs and humans attend an obedience class, or that you train your dog yourself before pursuing certification. Also visit a vet, and obtain any vaccinations or health certifications required by the organization with which you're pursuing certification.

The Evaluation Process:

When the prerequisites done, register for an evaluation with the certifying organization, and pay the appropriate fee. Read over the handbook, or instructions about the evaluation carefully so you're prepared for evaluation day. Evaluators will check the animal's temperament in various situations, and ensure you have the animal under control. Choosing a certifying organization with a chapter near you really helps, since it will make it easier to register for an evaluation that is not too far from home. After completing your initial evaluation, the certifying organization may have you attend your first few therapy sessions with your evaluator, so you and your pet can get feedback. Love on a Leash, for example, has its new members do 10 hours of supervised visits.

Chapter 4

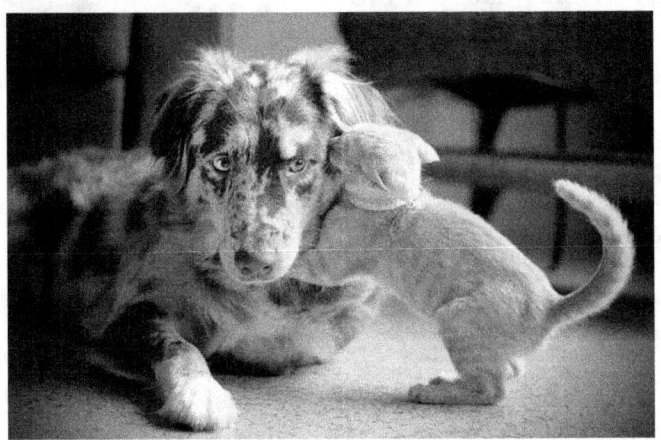

WHAT ARE THE SIDE EFFECTS OF PET THERAPY?

Patients who are allergic to animal dander may have reactions during pet therapy.

How Is Pet Therapy Administered?

The healthcare provider managing the patient's treatment administers pet therapy. A trained handler, often the pet's owner, takes the animal to every meeting. The animal and handler work under the provider's direction to help the patient reach pre-determined goals. In most cases, handlers worker as volunteers.

What Are the Steps of Pet Therapy?

The first step in pet therapy is the selection of a suitable animal. Many animal groups train, and connect volunteer owners and pets with health care providers.

Before an animal and its handler can participate in pet therapy, the team usually has to fulfill certain requirements.

This process typically includes:

-A physical examination of the animal to confirm that it is immunized and free of diseases.

-An obedience training course to ensure proper animal control.

-An instruction course to teach the trainer about patient interaction.

-An evaluation of the animal's temperament and behavior, and the handler.

-A certification from the sponsoring organization.

Once an animal-and-handler team is approved, animals are assigned for therapy based on patients' needs. The animal's type, breed, size, age, and natural behavior determine where it will be most helpful.

What are the Risks of Pet Therapy?

Some of the biggest risks of pet therapy involve safety and sanitation. Animals in pet therapy programs are typically screened for behavior and health. The animals' owners and handlers must also undergo training and evaluation to help ensure a positive experience.

While uncommon, human injury can occur when unsuitable animals are used. In addition, animals may suffer injury, or abuse when handled inappropriately.

In some cases, patients may become possessive of the animals helping them. This can result in problems with low self-esteem when unrealistic expectations aren't met. When an animal dies during pet therapy, patients may feel intense grief, or even guilt.

What is the Outlook After Pet Therapy?

The use and success of pet therapy is unique to each individual. Patients may have less anxiety during procedures when a pet is present. In rehabilitation, patients may be more motivated to practice their skills when working with a pet.

Patients suffering from sensory disabilities can communicate easily with a pet. This may encourage further human interaction with healthcare providers.

What Are the Results of Pet Therapy?

Patients in pet therapy may experience reduced cardiovascular reactions to stress. This is attributed to a process called "contact comfort." In this process, the unconditional human-animal bond that forms through touch is thought to induce relaxation.

Evidence of the physiological effects of pet therapy was found in a study of adult patients hospitalized with heart failure. Researchers credited pet therapy with improving levels of cardiopulmonary function, neurchormone levels, and anxiety.

Chapter 5

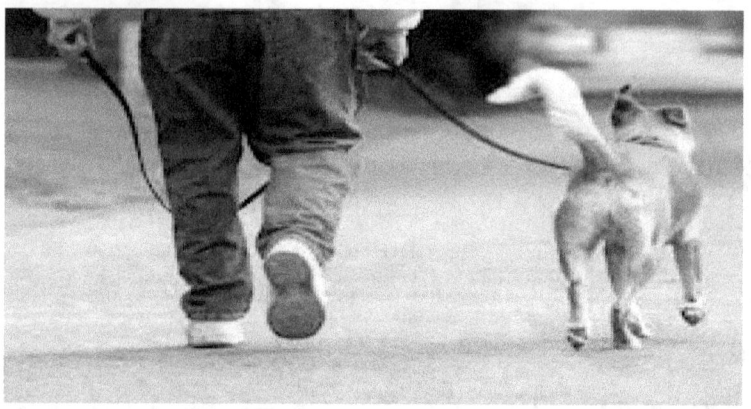

USING PET THERAPY TO HELP CONTROL YOUR MENTAL ILLNESS

Pet therapy is a broad term that includes animal-assisted therapy, and other animal-assisted activities. Animal-assisted therapy is a growing field that uses dogs, or other animals to help people recover from, or better cope with health problems, such as heart disease, cancer, and mental health disorders.

Animal-assisted activities, on the other hand, have a more general purpose, such as providing comfort and enjoyment for nursing home residents.

How does animal-assisted therapy work?

Imagine you're in the hospital. Your doctor mentions the hospital's animal-assisted therapy program, and asks if you'd be interested. You say yes, and your doctor arranges for someone to tell you more about the program. Soon after that, an assistance dog and its handler visit your hospital room. They stay for 10 to 15 minutes. You're invited to pet the dog, and ask the handler questions.

After the visit, you realize you're smiling. And you feel a little less tired, and a bit more optimistic. You can't wait to tell your family all about that charming canine. In fact, you're already looking forward to the dog's next visit.

Who can benefit from animal-assisted therapy?

Animal-assisted therapy can significantly reduce pain, anxiety, depression, and fatigue in people with a range of help the problems.

Children having dental procedures.

People receiving cancer treatment.

People in long-term care facilities.

People hospitalized with chronic heart failure.

Veterans with post-traumatic stress disorder.

And it's not only the ill person who reaps the benefits. Family members, and friends who sit in on animal visit say they feel better, too. Animals also can be taught to reinforce rehabilitative behaviors in patients, such as throwing a ball, or walking. Pet therapy is also being used in nonmedical settings, such as universities and community programs, to help people deal with anxiety and stress.

Animal-assisted therapy in action:

More than a dozen certified therapy dogs are part of Mayo Clinic's Caring Canines program. They make regular visit to various hospital departments, and even make special visits on request. The dogs are a welcome distraction, and help reduce the stress and anxiety that can accompany hospital visits.

Ways Your Pet Can Improve Your Mental Health:

A friend tells me when she is feeling down and weary, and can barely lift herself off the couch, her dog comes to her rescue. She cuddles with her, and they motivate her to get up, dress, and out the door for a walk, or some play time. Somehow her fur-baby even gets her to smile, no matter how miserable, or stressed she feels.

She is not alone. It turns out that all pets, not just therapy pets can help your mind, body and spirit.

Chapter 6

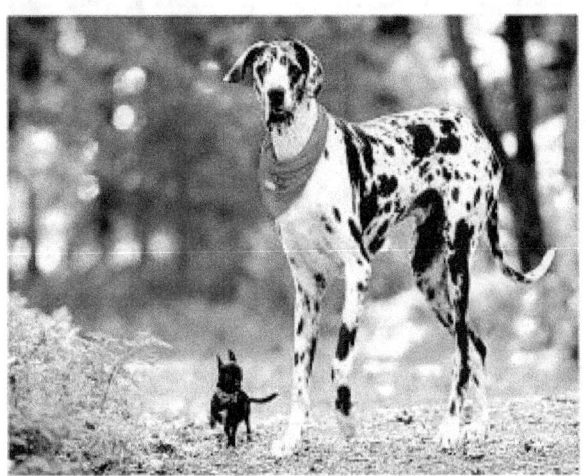

17 REASONS WHY TO USE PET THERAPY

1. **They get you outside:** Sun and fresh air elevate your mood, and the sun gives you an extra dose of vitamin D. Vitamin D exposure helps fight physical and mental conditions, including depression, cancer, obesity, and heart attacks. Also, when you go outside with your pet, you are engaging with nature. Try taking a moment to listen to the trees rustling, feel the wind rushing past, and sun upon your face. The sounds and feeling of nature can be incredibly calming.

2. **They get you moving**: Walking your dog, and engaging in out-doors activities like tossing a Frisbee gives you a natural energy boost, and allows you to let off steam. It also makes you more physically fit, strengthening your muscles and bones which helps not only with your body, but also your self-esteem. Studies have shown that animal owners both adults and children, have lower blood pressure, as well as lower

cholesterol and triglycerides, which may be in part attributed to the more active lifestyle pets promote. Pet owners also have been noted to have better circulation, and a lower risk of experiencing major cardiac issues. And when your body feels stronger, you are less susceptible to mental health issues.

3. **They lessen allergies and asthma, and build immunity**: This one may sound counterintuitive, but children who grow up in homes with furry friends are actually less likely to develop common allergies. Studies have shown that children who were exposed to two or more dogs or cats as babies ,were less than half as likely to develop allergies, including dust , grass, ragweed, and pet allergies, and were at a lower risk for asthma. Allergies can cause people to become lethargic, apathetic, and suffer from insomnia, which can make them more vulnerable to mental health issues, such as depression.

4. **Petting reduces stress.** Rhythmic petting, or grooming can be comforting to your dog or cat, and you. Concentrate on the texture of his soft fur, the warmth he radiates, and his deep breaths. When you connect with your pet, oxytocin, the hormone related to stress and anxiety relief, is released, helping to reduce blood pressure, and lower cortisol levels.

5. **They both distract you and keep you present**: Bring present, and engaged with your pet takes your thoughts off of the issues that are plaguing you. When you are fully in the moment, you are not worrying about the past or the future. It's just you and your pet. Another way to keep distracted and present with your furry friend is to take photos, or videos of his or her curt antics.

6. **They decrease loneliness.** If you don't like to be alone, pets can be great domestic companions. Often a pet is very intuitive, and will seek you out when you're feeling down, refusing to allow you to remain alone. Just make sure you can fully care for and love a pet before you take them home. Pets should not be used to fill a temporary void, and then pushed aside. A dog or cat is a long-term commitment, and it's not always easy, but if you are up to it, they can provide much love through the good times and the bad.

7. **They're great listeners:** You can talk to your pet about anything, your day, your hopes, and your dreams. You can practice a speech with them, lament about a breakup, or utter truths that you may be afraid to actually share with someone else. A dog or cat can be the perfect "person" to go to when you want to vent without any potential repercussions.

8. **They love you unconditionally**: Seeing their enthusiasm when you walk in can be an instant mood-lifting boost. Their tail wagging, tongue hanging out their mouth making it looks like they are smiling, the way their ears perk up. And listening to their grunts or purrs, they don't care if you just screwed up a deal at work, or bombed a test; they love you for being you, whatever that means on any given day their just happy to see you. They want to be around you, to love you, and be loved by you.

9. **They can decrease your isolation**: Dog parks allow for more opportunities for socialization for both your dog and you. Your dog makes friends pretty easily, and will break the ice so you can connect with new people, and perhaps set up future dog dates, hikes, or playtimes at local parks. Your little cutie can be an instant

conversation starter, and also a good way to get to know some of the people in your neighborhood.

10. **They can give you a purpose**: Having a pet to care for can give you a feeling of purpose, which can be crucial when you are feeling really down, and overwhelmed by negative thoughts. By caring for your pet, or another person or animal in need, you are focusing on something other than yourself and your life. Your good deeds, and your pet's positive response, will give you a feeling of instant gratification.

11. **They make you smile:** When your dog does cute things like rolling on their back, or putting a paw up on you arm, they can make you smile, which in turn triggers neurotransmitters to fire. These pet-time smiles can raise your serotonin and dopamine levels, which are nerve transmitters associated with calmness and happiness.

12. **Playing is fun:** With the grind of daily life, sometimes we forget to just let loose and have fun. Go ahead; wrestle, play catch, dance together, or just run around and act silly. Your dog will love you for it. So go ahead and have some fun with you pooch or feline friend: Have a ball, with a ball, or anything else, and you will both benefit from the pleasurable together time. And if you don't have a pet, or can't get one right now, you can volunteer at a shelter. There are many animals that can still benefit from your love, and you will feel the benefits too.

13. **The Health Benefits of Keeping Pets:** Pets, you can love and hate them at the same time. One moment they are sinking their teeth into you expensive shoes, and the next, they shower you with affection. But regardless of what they do and how you feel about

them, there is no denying that there are various health advantages of having a pet.

14. **Lower stress levels and blood pressure**: According to studies conducted at the University of Warwick interacting with pets (such as stroking them or playing with them) has the tendency to lower a person's blood pressure and relax them. In another study, stockbrokers with high blood pressure readings were asked to adopt a cat or a dog, and those who did were later found to have much lower blood pressure levels in stressful situations then those who did not adopt a pet. Of course, this will not work if you do not like animals, or are afraid of them "then they will probably cause more anxiety then they resolve.

15. **Recovery from illness:** Pets have been known to help people in astounding ways, but they have the greatest number of success stories with heart attack patients. Various studies show that patients who have suffered from a heart attack tend to live longer if they have a pet at home, and they are also less prone to heart disease than non-pet owners. Pets can also serve as a loyal support system to their bed-ridden owners, providing them with the comfort that results in a quicker recovery. In extreme cases, such as when a person is in a coma, surgeons have been recommended for a pet to be brought to the patient's bedside. While there is no real evidence to support this claim, there have been incidences when the pet's presence helped the patient awake from their coma. Dogs, in particular, have also been known to offer relief to Alzheimer's and Parkinson's patients.

16. **Improves social life:** Many domesticated animals are social creatures, and therefore provide much social interaction "whether it is a cat that curls up and fall

asleep on your lap, or a dog that follows you from room to room" a pet owner is very rarely alone. Pets also serve as great ice-breakers, or conversation starters among strangers, both inside and outside the home.

17. **Happiness:** It is often underestimated how much pets can influence our happiness; in many cases they have helped their owners deal with loss and hardships, even helping them fight depression. Some psychologists have even recommended the use of pets in therapy sessions, as petting a rabbit, or playing with a dog raises the serotonin levels in our brain. Being greeted by an energetic dog, or purring cat that is excited to see you can be very uplifting if you feel like your life just isn't going your way. This is why pets are also used in elderly homes to help individuals who feel lonely and isolated. Regardless of whether you face unemployment or divorce, your pet will continue to love you unconditionally; and it is precisely this love that keeps human beings healthy and happy.

<u>Conclusion</u>

Thank you again for choosing this book!

I hope this book was able to help you to understand how much your pet helps you to maintain a healthy life.

Consider your routine and schedule before committing to a pet. The last thing you need is added stress in your life, so select a pet that will work with your day-to-day schedule. Think about what the pet will require for care, and who will be responsible for that. The responsibility should be your child's, but what is the backup plan to care for the pet when your child is having a rough day? Again, a furry (or not-so-furry) friend that is low maintenance might work best for your family.

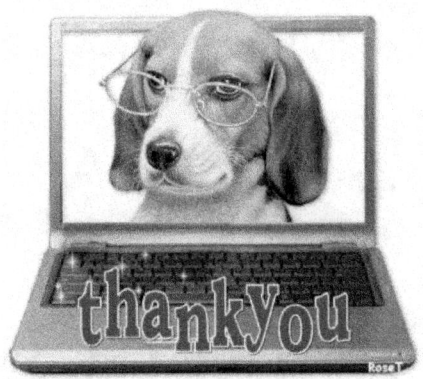

Finally, if you enjoyed this book, would you be kind enough to leave a review for this book on Amazon? It'd be greatly appreciated!

Thank you and good luck!

Preview Of 'INSECURE: Stop the Insecurity and Learn How to Overcome Jealousy and Build Self Esteem'

Chapter 1:

HOW TO STOP INSECURITY

Insecurity is not bad: People feel bad when they feel insecure because it's commonly believed that insecurity is a bad emotion that has no useful role in improving ones live. However when taking a closer look at the cause of insecurity you will find that insecurity is just a message sent by your brain trying to tell you one of the following things:

I am not sure of my ability to do this task.

I think I might be moving in the wrong direction or...

I might lose what I already have.

Insecurity is one of the strongest motivational forces

We human beings are either motivation by rewards or plain avoidance. Those who understand the fact that insecurity is just a message manage to completely eliminate their insecurities by providing reassurance to their minds. For example if you felt insecure about your job then improving your skills, taking additional courses, working harder and improving your CV will surely eliminate your insecurity. It's as if insecurity is the key driving force that pushes people to new achievements that they wouldn't have achieved otherwise if they didn't feel insecure. But sadly not all people manage to take advantage of the insecurity feelings, some people fail to understand the nature of the insecurity feelings and so live with them for extended periods of time or use quick fixes every now and then to temporary regulate their mood. Quick fixes can range from food, smoking, relationships up to drugs and self harm. The ultimate destination for people who use quick fixes is depression!

PATRICIA A. CARLISLE

INSECURE

Stop the Insecurity and Learn
how to Overcome Jealousy
and Build Self-Esteem

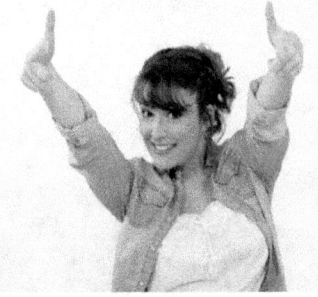

Go download and check out the rest of INSECURE: Stop the Insecurity and Learn how to Overcome Jealousy and Build Self-Esteem on amazon.com

Check Out My Other Books

Below you'll find some of my other popular books that are popular on Amazon and Kindle as well. Alternatively, you can visit my author page on Amazon to see other work done by me. (https://amazon.com/author/patriciacarlisle)

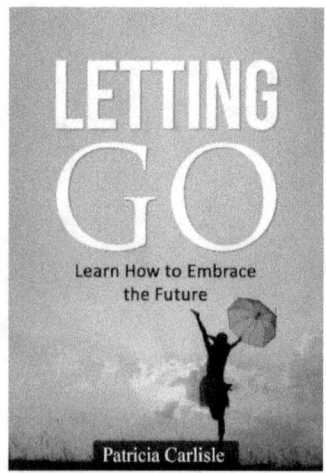

LETTING GO: Learn How to Embrace the Future.

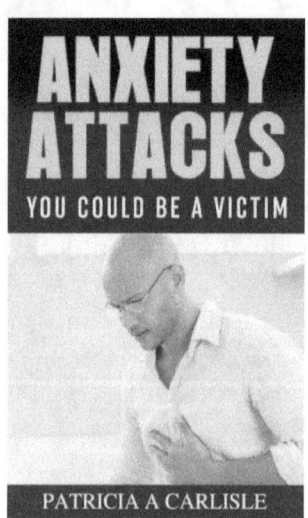

ANXIETY ATTACKS: YOU COULD BE A VICTIM

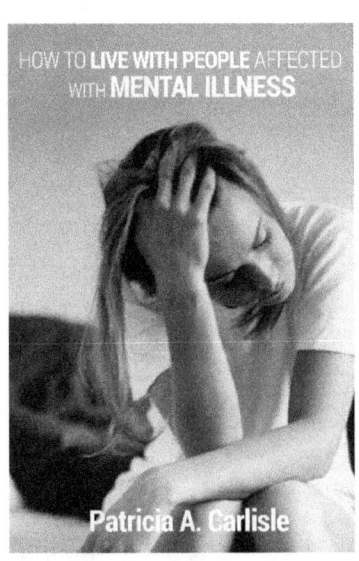

HOW TO LIVE WITH PEOPLE AFFECTED WITH MENTAL ILLNESS.

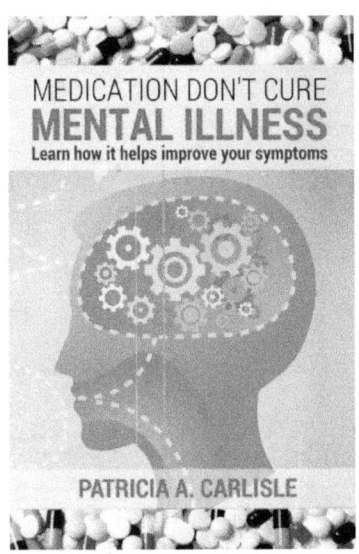

MEDICATION DON'T CURE MENTAL ILLNESS: Learn how it helps improve your symptoms.

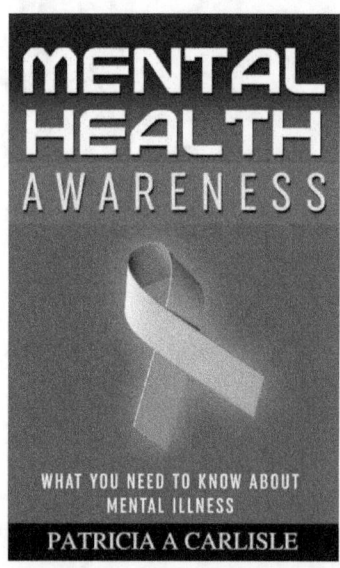

MENTAL HEALTH AWARNESS: WHAT YOU NEED TO KNOW ABOUT MENTAL ILLNESS.

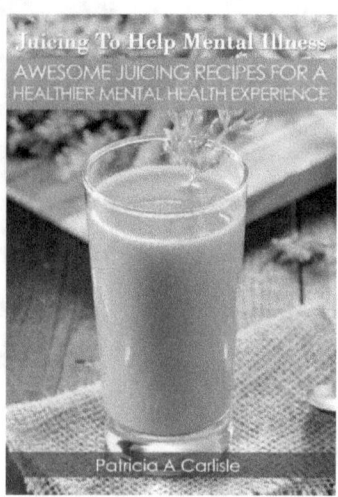

Juicing To Help Mental Illness. Awesome Juicing recipes for a healthier mental Health Experience.

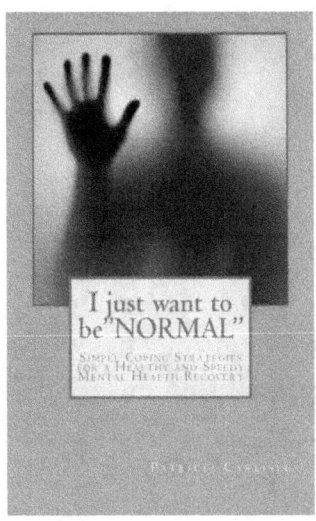

I just want to be "NORMAL" simple coping STRATEGIES For a Healthy and Speedy mental health Recovery

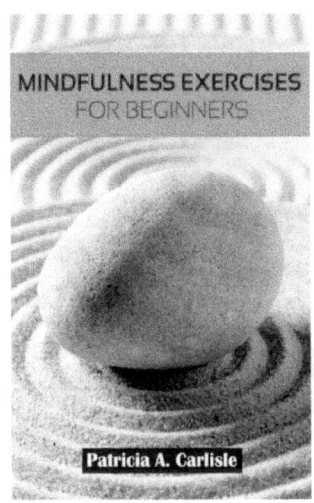

MINDFULNESS EXERCISES FOR BEGINNERS.

You can simply search for these titles on the Amazon website to find them.

BONUS: SUBSCRIBE TO THE FREE BOOK

Beginners Guide to Yoga & Meditation

"Stressed out? Do You Feel Like The World Is Crashing Down Around You? Want To Take A Vacation That Will Relax Your Mind, Body And Spirit? Well this Easy To Read Step By Step

E-Book Makes It All Possible!"

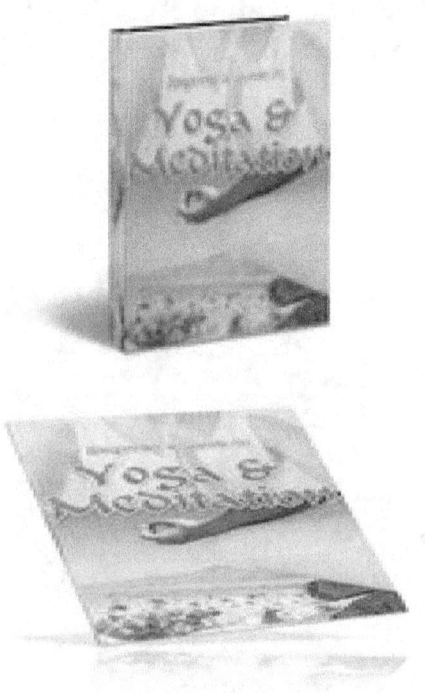

Instructions on how to join our mailing list, and receive a free copy of "Yoga and Meditation" can be found in any of my Kindle eBooks.

NOTES

NOTES

NOTES

NOTES

NOTES

NOTES

www.ingramcontent.com/pod-product-compliance
Lightning Source LLC
Chambersburg PA
CBHW061928280526
45787CB00004B/1530